Coconut Oil

Enjoy Health and Beauty Benefits By Using Oil from Nature's "Tree of Life"

RON KNESS

Contents

Disclaimer

This publication is for informational purposes only and is not intended as medical advice. Medical advice should always be obtained from a qualified medical professional for any health conditions or symptoms associated with them.

Every possible effort has been made in preparing and researching this material. We make no warranties with respect to the accuracy, applicability of its contents or any omissions.

See your healthcare professional before starting any diet, health or exercise program!

Introduction

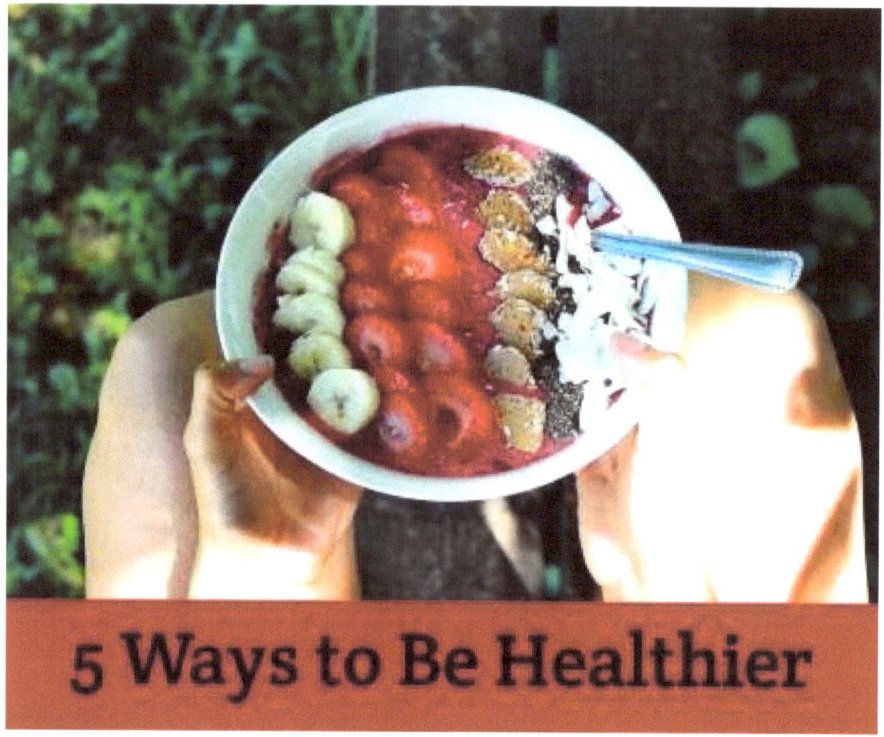

5 Ways to Be Healthier

5 Steps to Being Healthier

If you want to live a healthier lifestyle, there are a lot of ways to do that. The following tips are not only going to include some of the methods you have heard countless times, like diet and exercise, but also incorporating some natural health remedies into your life.

Incorporate Coconut Oil Into Your Life

Coconut oil is one of the best natural remedies for health in general, helping for so many different things. This is why it is at the top of the list. Try to incorporate more of it into your life, from adding it to your diet, to rubbing it on your skin or using it on your hair and nails.

Coconut oil is natural, but you do want to choose the organic or virgin kind so it doesn't come with any additives. There are a lot of healthy snacks and meals you can prepare that use coconut oil.

Drink Lots of Water

Drinking more water is crucial if you want to be a healthier person. You should try to drink at least 8-10 glasses of water a day, more if your doctor recommends it based on your needs or your weight. If you sweat a lot during the day, you should be drinking more water to replenish those fluids. Try to choose a fun cup or bottle as this can encourage you to drink more water. You might also want to try fruit-infused water.

Follow a Healthy Diet

This might not be what you wanted to hear, but your diet is a big part of being healthy, whether you are losing weight or not. Even if you aren't trying to lose weight, you should always focus on proper nutrition. It is good for overall health, and even helps with things like your digestion, reducing headaches and migraines, and avoiding more serious diseases later in life. Focus on a well-balanced meal every time you eat with enough protein, carbs, fruits, veggies, and whole grains.

Get Your Body Moving

Exercise doesn't have to be hitting the gym for 3 hours every day, but you should definitely keep your body moving. Every day, try to get up and get some type of exercise.

On busy workdays, take your afternoon break outside where you walk around the building a few times, or go for a hike over the weekend to really get your blood pumping. Take your dogs on an extra walk in the evening, or ride bikes with your kids. There are a lot of ways to get more exercise without trying very hard.

Go Outside

You may be missing vitamin D, which you can get from the sunshine. If you work indoors, it might be hard for you to force yourself outside for those natural rays. However, if you're adding in exercise, this makes it a lot easier.

Types of Coconut Oils

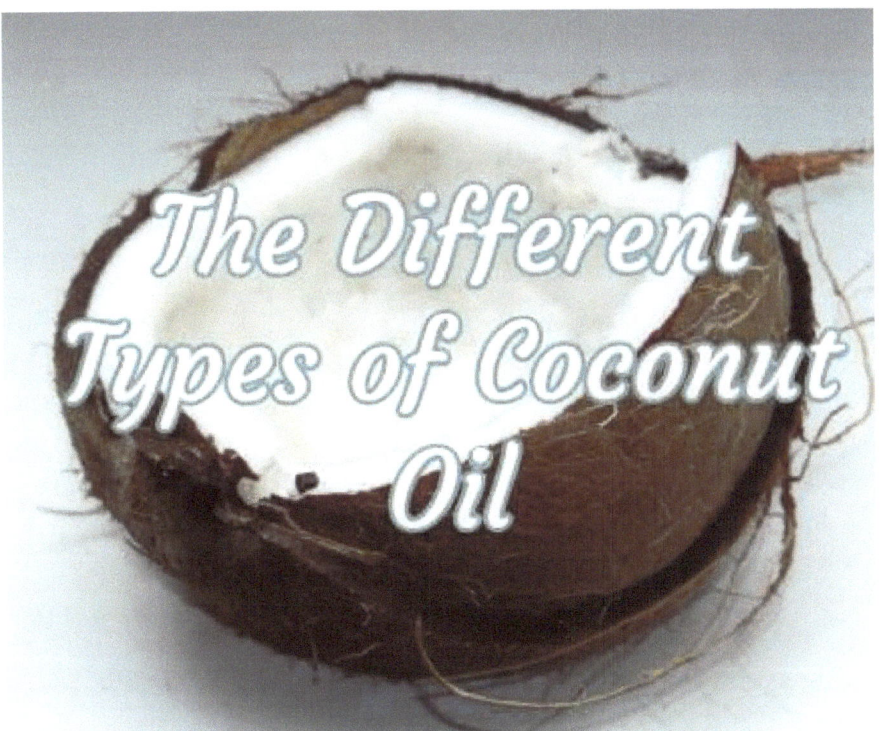

When you begin looking at the health benefits to using more coconut oil in your life, you may notice that the store has a lot of different types. It is important to understand what type of coconut oil you need in order for it to be most beneficial. Here are some different types of coconut oil to be aware of.

Organic Coconut Oil

The first type of coconut oil you want to be sure you get is organic coconut oil. This means that the coconuts themselves were grown without any pesticides or other chemicals.

This shouldn't be the only label you look for, but when you want it to be as natural as possible, look for the words organic on the label. If you are in the United States, this will usually need to be "USDA Organic" to qualify.

Unrefined Coconut Oil

Another label that you might see when you go shopping for your coconut oil is either refined or unrefined. A good way to look at it is that refined coconut oil is more processed than unrefined coconut oil, so it is best to go with the jar that says unrefined on the label. When coconut oil is refined, it means that a lot of the flavor of the coconut is removed from the oil by choosing a higher smoke point for preparing the oil. This is done for people who like the benefits of coconut oil, but don't want the flavor. However, this process keeps it from being fresh and raw.

Virgin or Extra Virgin Coconut Oil

You will frequently see that extra virgin or virgin coconut oil is recommended for food, drinks, or personal use. Pay close attention to the label of the coconut oil you purchase so that you get the right variety. You aren't paying much attention to the difference between virgin or extra virgin coconut oil, but that at least one of these terms are used. It is not like olive oil where there is a difference between these. It simply means it is lighter than pure coconut oil, which is needed in some circumstances.

You may also notice other types of coconut oil, like cold pressed or processed coconut oil. The use and recipe for your DIY purposes will determine what type of coconut oil to use.

However, in general, you should go with the unrefined organic coconut oil, often looking for it to say raw, virgin, or extra virgin on the label.

How to Get Coconut Oil to Not Harden

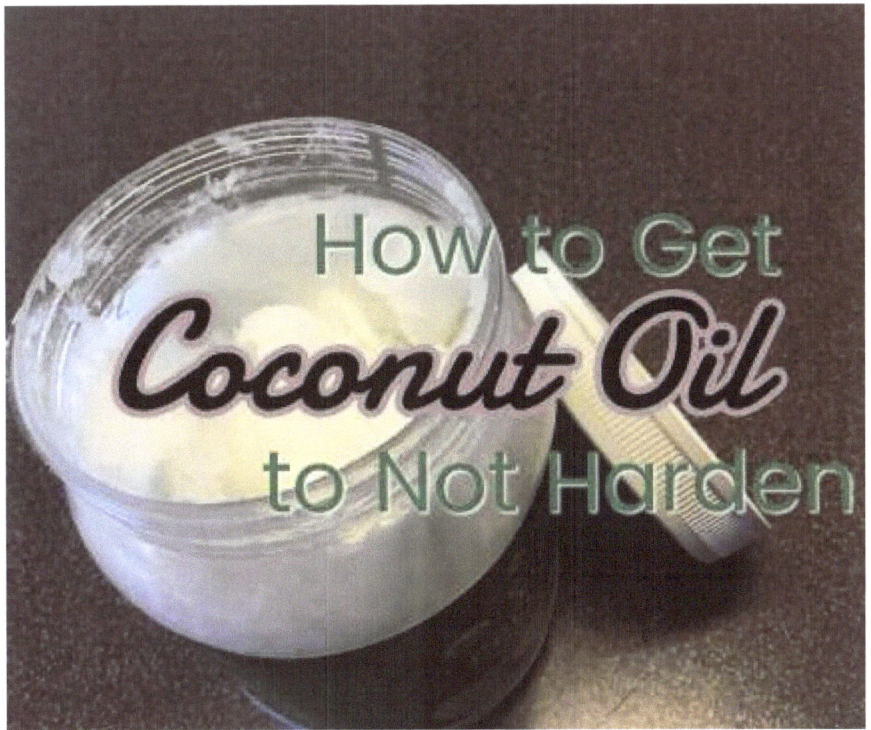

Coconut oil can be used for many different things, from cooking with it as a healthier cooking oil option, to using it on your hair. However, the oil itself does not come in a liquid like olive oil or canola oil. Instead, it is a thick substance that first needs to be softened. However, there are some ways to keep it from hardening completely.

Combine it With Other Oils

As you probably know, other types of oil remains as a liquid. You can combine your coconut oil with these other oils, keep it stored in a bottle or container, and keep it as a liquid. This does require using the other ingredients along with your coconut oil, but they can all be beneficial for you. A good option is to combine it with olive oil, making sure it is 1 part coconut oil and 1 part olive oil. This is safe for your skin and very soft and moisturizing. You can also try adding in some essential oils and kosher salt to turn it into a scrub that will never harden completely.

Leave it in a Hot Environment

Another good way you can keep your coconut oil from hardening if you want to keep it more of a liquid consistency is by storing it in a hot environment. Unlike cooking oils like vegetable oil or olive oil, you don't actually have to keep the coconut oil stored in a cold, dry climate to keep it from spoiling. Coconut oil can handle different environments, it just might not remain fresh for quite as long. If you tend to need the coconut oil as liquid most of the time and don't want to worry about actually warming it up, then keep it in an area of your home that is warmer, or even near a window where the sun will shine down on the container.

Warm the Coconut Oil Quickly

Warming coconut oil is actually really simple to do and doesn't require even using a microwave, which is not recommended. If you are not able to keep the coconut oil in a way that keeps it a liquid, then you can simply rub the small container between your hands. Keep rubbing it until it starts to soften.

Another method is to use a double boiler, with water in the bottom pan, then the container of coconut oil in the top. This also takes just a few minutes.

Common Mistakes Made With Coconut Oil

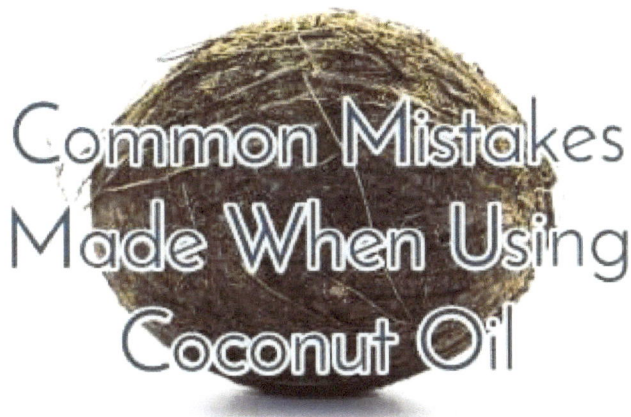

Adding more coconut oil into your diet or using on your skin or hair is a wonderful way to benefit from it, but there are also some mistakes people tend to make. Make sure if you decide to use more coconut oil on a daily basis, you do not make these common mistakes.

Allowing Mold to Grow

It is normal to have multiple jars of coconut oil in your home and use it often. The problem with this is that each jar might take a while to use completely, which means a lot of humidity and wet hands going into the jar consistently over time can lead to mildew and even mold. You definitely don't want to be using coconut oil that has started to grow mold on it. A good way to prevent this is by either keeping just one jar in your home and using it up before buying another one, or just making sure your hands are always dry when using it. If you use it on wet hair or after a shower, be careful about scooping it from the jar and dry your hands first.

Using it on Color-Treated Hair

This is a common mistake mostly because there aren't enough warning out there. You need to be really careful about using too much coconut oil on color-treated hair, as it might cause the color to fade prematurely. This doesn't mean that you can never use it on your dyed hair, but that you need to be more careful. You should only use it about once a week or so, and a smaller amount than others would use. You also might not want to leave it in your hair for as long. Test a small section underneath your hair first to make sure it doesn't cause a major change in your hair color.

Letting it Get Too Close to Your Eyes

You need to be really careful when you are putting the coconut oil near your eyes, particularly if you are using it as a carrier oil with essential oils. Many people like to apply coconut oil to their face as a moisturizer or combine it with essential oils into a headache balm to rub on the forehead.

This works great, but be really careful not to get it in your eyes. Coconut oil will burn, but essential oils can cause even more serious problems.

Potential Side Effects of Coconut

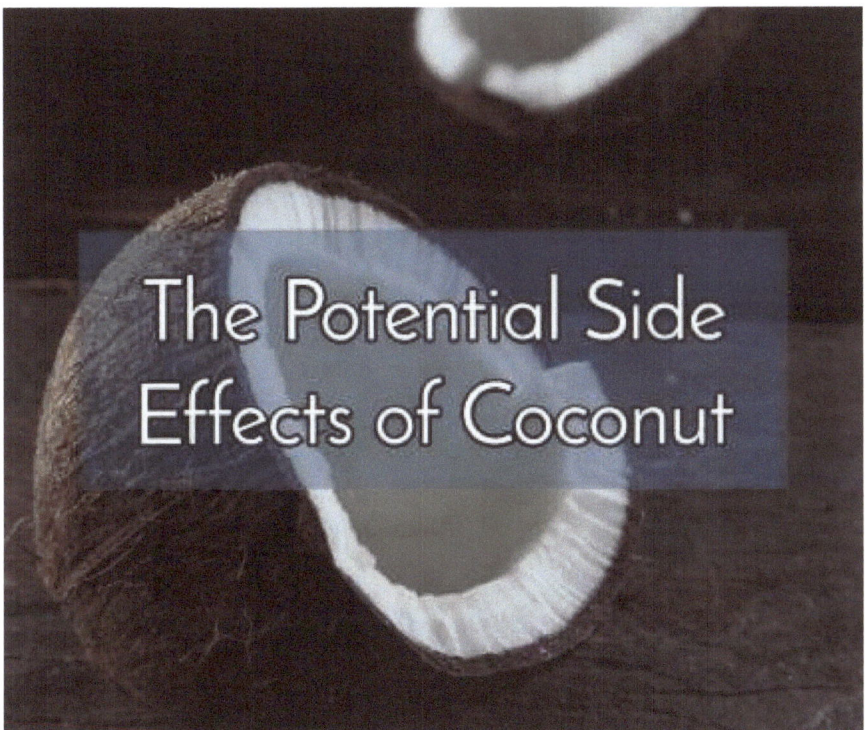

When it comes to natural health remedies, coconut and coconut oil specifically is often recommended. It can be used on bug bites, to help with arthritis pain, help your hair grow, clean your teeth, and even be used as deodorant. While it is safe to use for most people and consume if you cook with it, you need to be aware of some minor side effects before you start using it.

It Can Increase Your Cholesterol

This is something to be aware of if you are consuming the coconut oil by cooking with it, instead of just using it on your skin or hair. While it is considered a healthy fat and something that is good to have in your body, there is such thing as having too much of it. You should still consider property dietary guidelines and not put it in absolutely everything you cook during the day. If you do, you might accidentally raise your cholesterol levels.

Some People Have Allergic Reactions

While this is not super common, it is definitely something you need to be aware of. Coconut oil is generally safe for most people, but some individuals have more sensitive skin and might have a bad reaction to it. For example, newborn babies and elderly people have thin, more sensitive skin, and might not react well to the coconut oil. It is also possible that someone simply has an allergic reaction to it, especially if they don't respond well to coconut flakes or coconut milk when eating or drinking. It is best to test a small area of the skin or have just a small amount of oil in food to test the reactions before using it more substantially.

It Occasionally Causes Diarrhea Symptoms

You should be aware that when consuming a lot of coconut oil, it might cause diarrhea in some people. Coconut oil is often recommended for people with digestion issues, including those who struggle with constipation. It works great for this purpose, but if you consume a lot of coconut oil and don't have digestion issues, it might do the opposite and actually give you diarrhea.

For this reason, you should start with just small amounts of coconut oil whether taking it straight or making food or drinks with the oil. If your body handles it fine without diarrhea or other negative reactions, then you can start consuming it a little more often. The same goes for using this oil on your skin.

Could Coconut Oil Be the New Fountain of Youth?

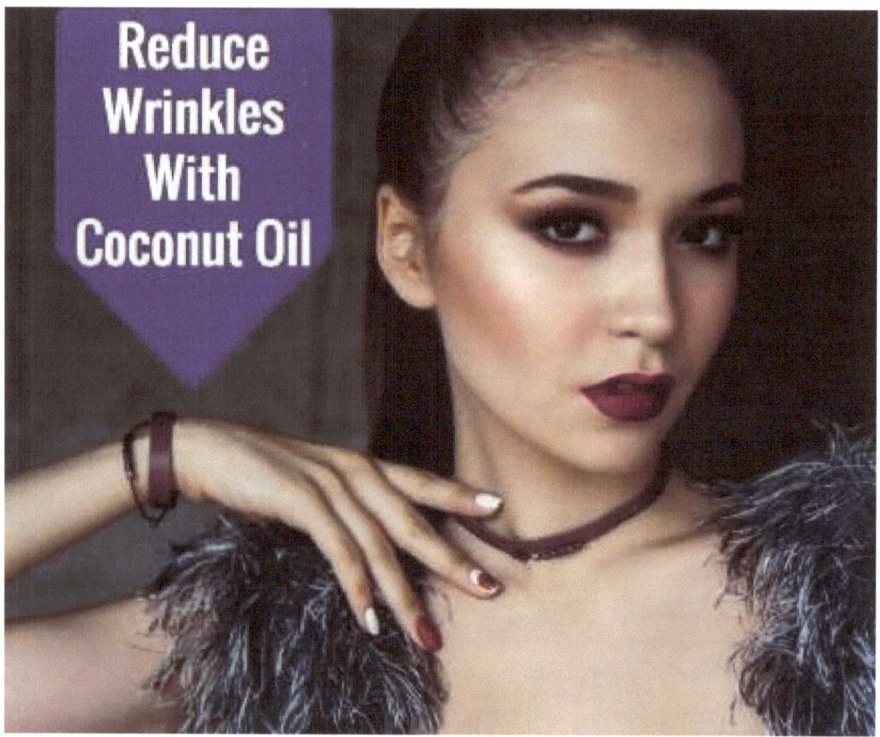

Coconut is often considered a miracle cure because of all the different ways it can benefit you. One great way to use coconut is by helping with anti-aging in a more natural way. Get rid of the expensive Botox and harsh chemicals of your store-bought cream and try these different coconut oil anti-aging tips.

Apply Coconut Oil to Your Wrinkles

The first way to use coconut for anti-aging purposes is simply to apply coconut oil on all your fine lines and wrinkles. Try to do this daily, preferably during your nighttime routine.

This makes it easy for you to remember and allows the oil to work overnight. Keep a container of virgin, organic coconut on your bedside table and rub it on your wrinkles or lines before bed. You don't need to rinse it off, so just use it like you would lotion or moisturizer. Keep applying it each day, but also try to consume some coconut in your meals and drinks as well.

Take a Coconut Oil Bath

Here is another great way to use coconut oil for your anti-aging purposes, particularly on your wrinkles and fine lines. The bath is a good option when you don't want to mess around with creams and lotions that you have to apply to your skin and leave a messy residue. All you need to do bring a jar of coconut oil into the bathtub with you. When you get in the bath, before sitting down in the water, apply the coconut oil to your skin. Let it absorb until dry, then soak into the bath and it will keep working its magic. After your bath, your skin will be soft and you don't have to rinse of the coconut oil.

Combine the Oil With Milk and Eggs

This is another concoction you can make if you want to use coconut oil for anti-aging purposes. The egg whites are really good for tightening your skin in order to prevent further wrinkles, while the milk helps to hydrate the skin and make it glow and look more youthful. Make sure you are only using the egg whites, and not yellow yolks from your eggs. You need to combine equal parts coconut oil and honey, then 1 egg white and the same amount of milk as you did with the coconut oil and honey. About a tablespoon of each works good. Mix it together in a bowl, then massage the mixture onto your skin. Store anything left in a small container.

Beauty In the Bedroom

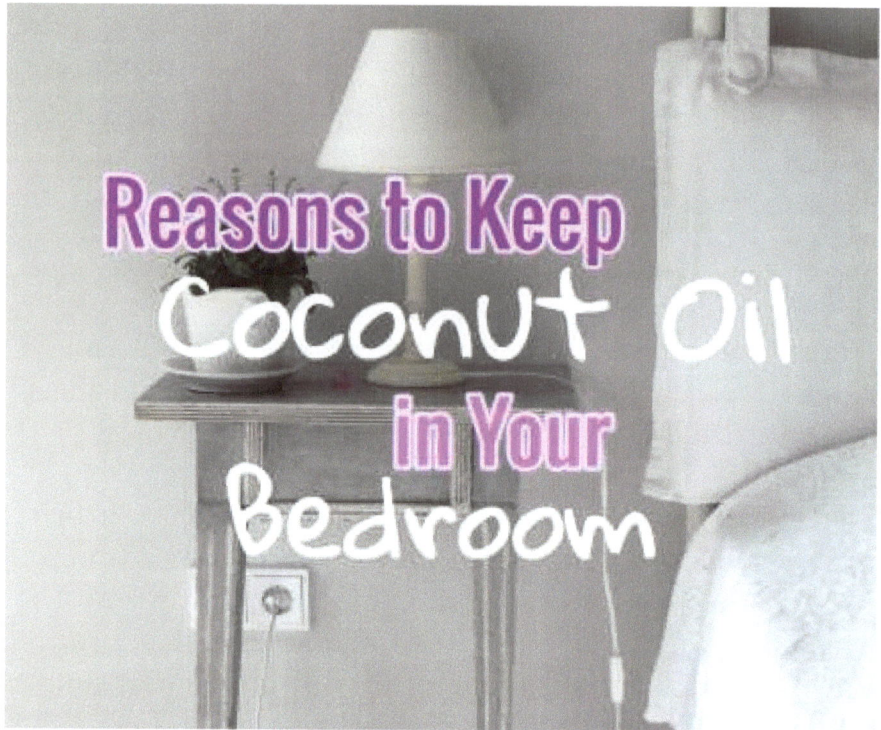

Coconut oil is often considered a miracle cure, as it can help with so many things. People use it for shiny hair and soft skin, to clean their teeth and freshen their breath, and add it to their food for loads of health benefits. It is something you should always have in the house, including your bedroom. Here are some different reasons to keep coconut oil in the bedroom.

You Have Instant Moisturizer

While there are a lot of different DIY products you can make by using coconut oil as an ingredient, you don't necessarily need some fancy balm or concoction just to get good use out of it.

All you really need to do is keep a container of it in your bedroom on your nightstand, then use a little bit in the palm of your hand whenever you need some moisturizer. It is a great option for ashy elbows, dry ankles, or to moisturize any part of your skin when you're in a pinch.

It Works For Those Itchy Dogs

This is something not a lot of people think about when they are in bed. If you have a dog that struggles with itchy skin, no matter what you do, then you know how frustrating it is to watch your dog uncomfortable and scratching all night. Plus the sound of your dog scratching constantly can disrupt your sleep quite a bit. To help your dog and yourself, keep some coconut oil in the bedroom that you can apply to your dog's skin before bed. It is safe to use on dogs and will help a lot with the itchy skin, plus help take care of the redness and irritation. You should test a small area first to make sure it doesn't give your dog any negative reactions.

You Can Remove Your Eye Makeup

If you forget to wash your face before bed and don't want to head back to the bathroom, you can simply keep some coconut oil in your bedroom to remove your eye makeup quickly and easily. Just keep a jar of coconut oil and some cotton balls in your bedroom.

Coconut Oil is the Perfect Night Cream

Your face is not the only place you might want to moisturize at night. You can also use your coconut oil on the bedside table as a night cream, such as a hand cream to wake up to soft hands, or even on your feet if you also like to moisturize them before bed. Having it in the bedroom makes it really easy to use on any dry skin.

3 Foot Cream Recipes

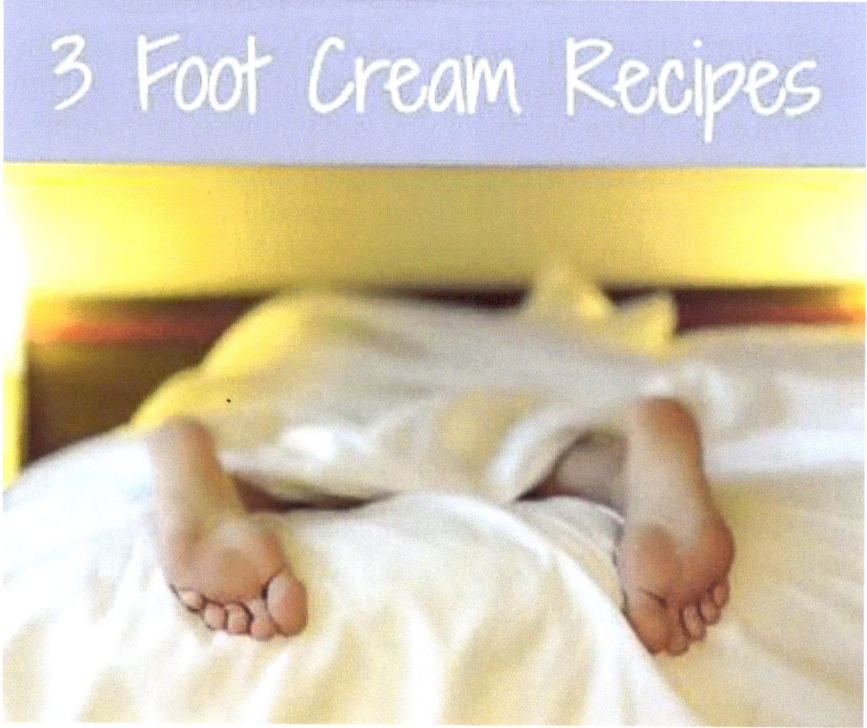

One of the areas of the body that often gets overlooked is the feet. People often forget to take good care of their feet, ignoring the rough, callused edges. However, if you want to have soft, beautiful feet, then a foot cream might be in order. These foot cream recipes are all natural, many of which use coconut oil.

Peppermint Foot Cream

This is definitely one of the more popular foot cream recipes, and can also be made with coconut oil. Peppermint in general is often used with foot crème because peppermint has a storing scent that is great for deodorizing your feet and helping the fresh smell to last a lot longer. For this DIY foot cream, you want to use coconut oil in its solid form, aloe vera gel, and peppermint essential oil. You can also add in other essential oils, but be careful about combining too many different scents together. You just need to whip the ingredients together to get a cream consistency, then make sure you store it properly.

Shea Butter and Beeswax Foot Cream

Here is another excellent recipe for a coconut oil foot cream. This one will use extra ingredients that provide even more softness and moisture for your feet. This includes adding some shea butter, which is so soft on your skin, and beeswax that is grated. You will also add in some coconut oil and olive oil, along with your choice of essential oils. Vanilla is a really good scent for this type of coconut oil, but as with many other foot creams, you can also add in a few drops of peppermint essential oils.

Coconut Lavender Foot Cream

If you want a foot cream that not only moisturizes your feet, but can also provide a relaxing and soothing experience, lavender is the perfect option. To make this type of foot cream, you will still need to start with your coconut oil, usually a couple tablespoons of it, then add about ½ cup of olive oil.

Combine this in a bowl with the same amount of beeswax pastilles, and add in as many drops of lavender essential oil as you want. You should start with 5 drops, mix it, then smell it to see if it is strong enough. Add about 5 drops at a time until you're happy. For this much cream, 15-20 is usually enough.

You can also make a plain foot cream that just uses coconut oil with something cream based, or you can whip the oil to make a cream consistency, then apply it to your feet.

How to Get Rid of Split Ends

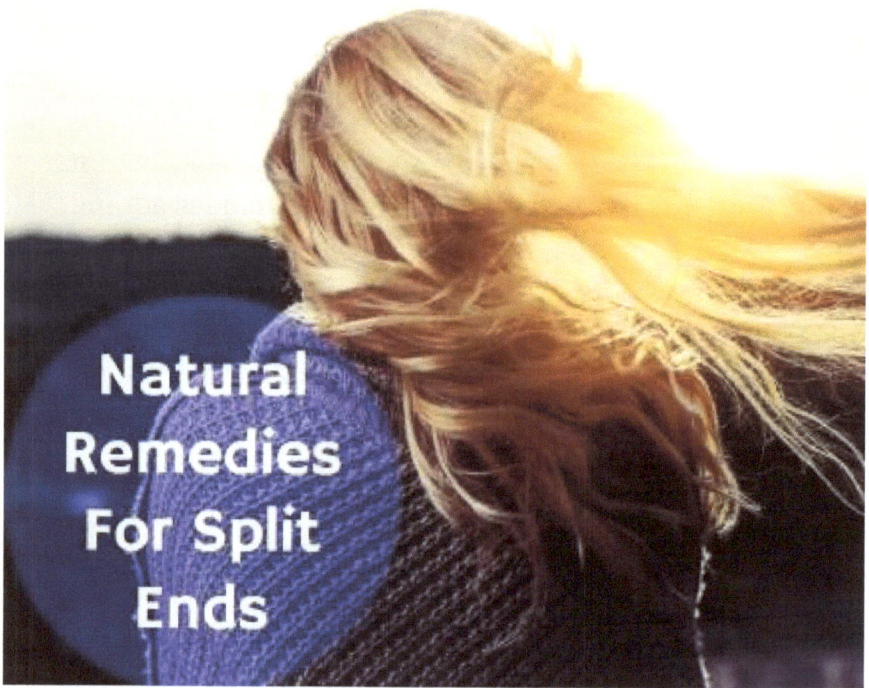

Split ends can be frustrating to deal with, especially when you don't want to keep trimming your hair.

However, if they are not too severe, there might be some other things you can do first. Here are some more natural ways of taking care of your split ends.

Try Using Coconut Oil

A really great way to help treat your split ends in a more natural way than just trimming them is by using coconut oil directly on the split ends. Coconut oil has tons of benefits, particularly for your hair and skin. Many people just use it to moisturize their hair or use it as a hair mask by leaving it in overnight and rinsing out the oil in the morning. You can do this, but really just applying it to your ends is going to help with those pesky split ends. You want to first towel dry your hair after you have washed it. Grab a small amount of coconut oil right from the jar, then work it through your hair, just applying to the middle through to the ends. Avoid applying it near your scalp as you already have natural oils there. Wrap your hair in a towel and then rinse it out in about 30-60 minutes. Do this about once a week or so and your split ends will thank you.

Add a Hot Oil Conditioner

Another way to reduce your split ends by conditioning is by using a hot oil conditioner. This can still work with your coconut oil, or you can use olive oil in its place. Hot oil treatments should not be done every day, but instead about once a week or so. They might not get rid of current split ends, but they can definitely keep them from getting worse. Doing this on a routine basis is going to help you keep them away for longer stretches of time without having to constantly cut your hair. To make your own hot oil treatment, just heat up some coconut oil or other type of oil for about 15-20 seconds in the microwave.

Massage it onto your scalp and through your hair, leaving it up for up to an hour. You can then rinse it out and wash your hair with shampoo.

Use an Egg Hair Mask

One more way to utilize coconut oil and other healthy oils in your hair is by creating a hair mask using both eggs and the oil. You can use eggs and coconut oil, add in olive oil, or any combination depending what you have. Adding in some honey can also be really great for your hair. With this type of hair mask, just leave it in for about 20 minutes, then rinse it out with cool water.

How to Use Coconut Oil Overnight

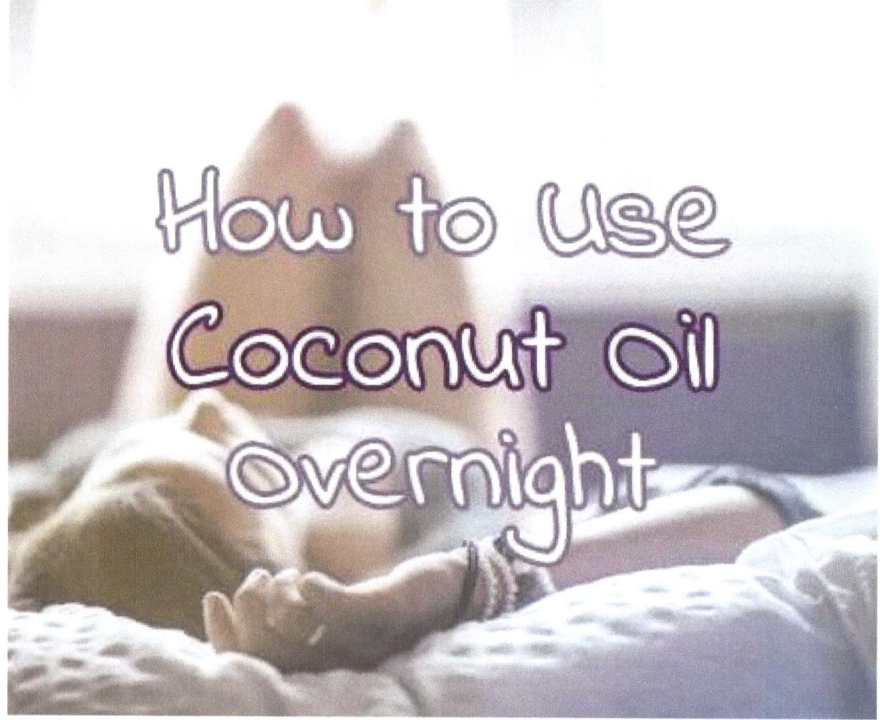

If you want to use coconut oil for soft, healthy, luxurious hair, there are a few ways to do that. You could add some coconut oil to your hair as a mask and leave it in for an hour before rinsing it out, or you can apply it before a heat treatment to protect your hair. Another good option is to create a mask you use overnight, which really allows the coconut to soak into your hair follicles. Here are some ways to use the coconut oil overnight.

Why Coconut Oil Helps Your Hair

First of all, you might be curious about why so many people recommend using coconut oil for your hair. There are a few different reasons it can be so great for healthy hair. This includes moisturizing it and getting rid of dryness, having a lightweight moisturizer, helping with split ends, and the fact that coconut oil contains a lot of proteins and nutrients that other hair oils don't have. It can also be really great for getting rid of all that buildup on your scalp that ultimately leads to dandruff.

Directions For Using it

Now you can learn exactly how to use the coconut oil overnight for your hair. Keep in mind that if you keep it in your bedroom, it might not be in a liquid consistency. The jars of coconut oil keep it solid, but it can still be used in your hair. What you want to do is just get some coconut oil into the palm of your hands, and rub it in between your hands carefully (don't make a mess!), to warm it up enough to run through your hair. You want to have about 2-3 tablespoons each night for your hair mask. If you keep it in the kitchen, you might prefer placing the jar in a pot on the stove for just a minute or so until it softens enough.

Just take the softened coconut oil and run it through your hair. It can be helpful to grab a comb after you have applied it to your hair and comb it through to get evenly throughout your hair. Leave it in your hair overnight. You may want to cover your pillow with a towel or wrap your hair for the night.

With these simple tips, you will be on your way to having beautiful, soft, luxurious hair just by applying the coconut oil overnight.

Use Coconut Oil for Healing

Coconut Oil For Natural Sunburn Relief

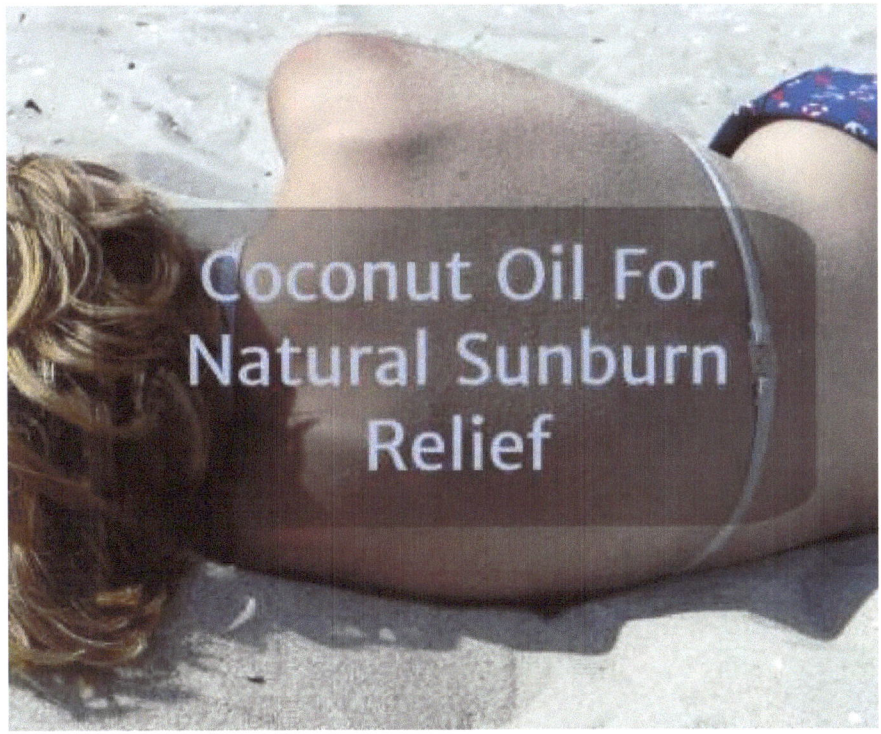

If you are prone to getting your skin burnt, you know how important it is to protect it on a regular basis with sunscreen. However, you may still get a sunburn even if you remembered to put on sunscreen, especially if you have fair skin. Here is a way to use coconut oil as a natural sunburn relief.

Create a Natural Sunburn Balm

The first thing you can do with your coconut oil when using it for a natural sunburn relief is by making a balm.

This is ideally going to use coconut oil, along with some essential oils that have a soothing effect. Lavender essential oil is really great for this purpose, but you can also try using chamomile as well. You want to combine the coconut oil with lavender essential oils, along with some aloe vera that comes straight from the plant. This is going to provide a lot of relief for your sunburn.

How to Use the Natural Sunburn Balm

When you have created your natural sunburn relief balm, you will then need to know how to use it. The consistency should be similar to regular sunscreen, though it might be a little bit thinner than what you are used to. It is important to keep two things in mind; you need to ensure you have rubbed it on all areas of skin that will be exposed to the sun, and you re-apply it on a regular basis. Since it is made of only natural ingredients, you shouldn't need to wash your hands after applying it to your skin. That is one of the main benefits of making a natural sunburn relief balm instead of using regular sunscreen. It also smells great!

Other Tips For Using Coconut Oil

If you have a sunburn, keep in mind that you might want to mix your coconut oil with something else to dilute the strength. For example, you can combine the coconut oil with vitamin E oil, which helps to protect your skin from the sun's UV rays, but can also moisturize your skin. This is great because there are so many added benefits, but it is also going to relieve your sunburn. If your sunburn is 2nd degree or higher, which will be bright red with blistering, you should consult a doctor before you put anything on it. The doctor might prefer you use aloe vera gel only.

How to Make a Headache Balm with Coconut

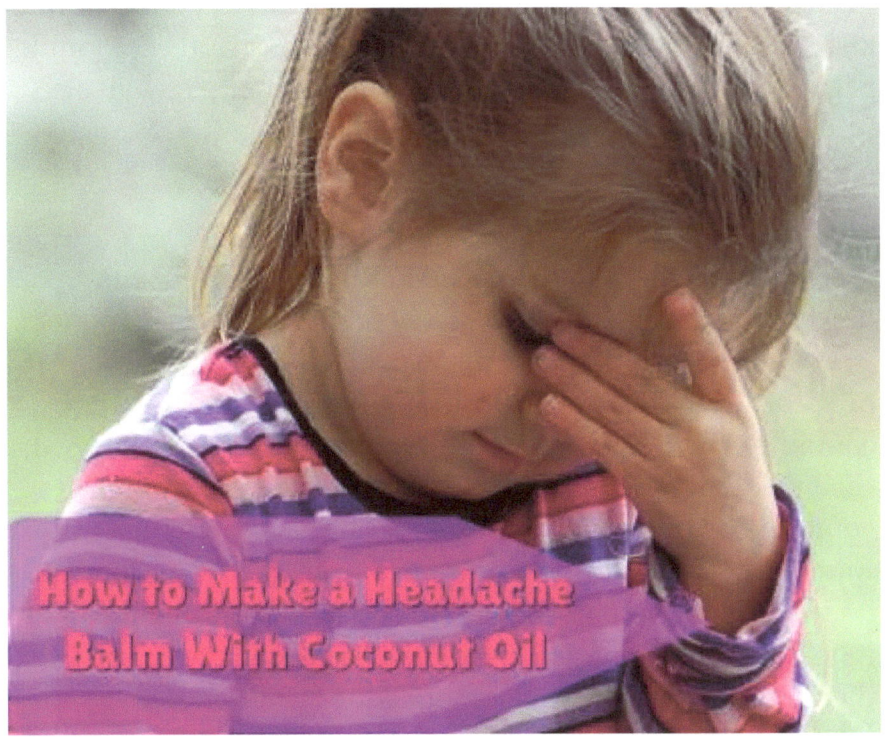

Headaches are common, but that doesn't mean it isn't really frustrating to experience them. While there are a lot of over-the-counter pain relievers that work great for headaches, if you get them chronically, you might not want to take medication constantly. A better option is to use a natural remedy such as coconut oil. Here is more information about making a headache balm with coconut oil.

Gather Your Ingredients

The first step to making the headache balm is to gather the required ingredients. For this type of DIY product, you will first need organic and raw coconut oil, making sure you don't choose coconut oil that has preservatives or weird chemicals.

27

Once you have that, you also want to choose some essential oils. These are up to you, but choose ones known to help with headaches, such as lavender and frankincense. Peppermint is also good for both headaches and migraines, and chamomile is good if you want it to help you sleep as well. You will also need a container for the balm and a double boiler.

Make the Headache Balm

Now that you have all the necessary ingredients for the headache balm, it is time to start preparing it. What you want to do is first get your coconut oil to melt, since it is probably in its solid form. You can do this by putting the container or a small amount of coconut oil into a glass bowl, then placing it in the top of a double boiler. You can make your own by putting a medium pot on the stove with a little water in it, then putting a bowl on top of the pot (as long as it doesn't fall into the pot), and the coconut oil in that bowl. Let it heat up for a few minutes to melt the coconut oil. You will then remove it from the heat and add in your chosen essential oils. Mix it well and pour it into a container and let it cool. Once it is cool, you are ready to use the balm.

Using Your Headache Balm

Once you are done making the coconut oil headache balm, you will need to learn how to use it. This works best when applied to your forehead shortly after you start getting a headache. It is going to soak into the skin, and that combined with the scent from the calming essential oils, it can help relieve pain as a result of the headache. You can also rub some on a damp washcloth, and rest that on your forehead to find relief.

Use Coconut Oil With Essential Oils

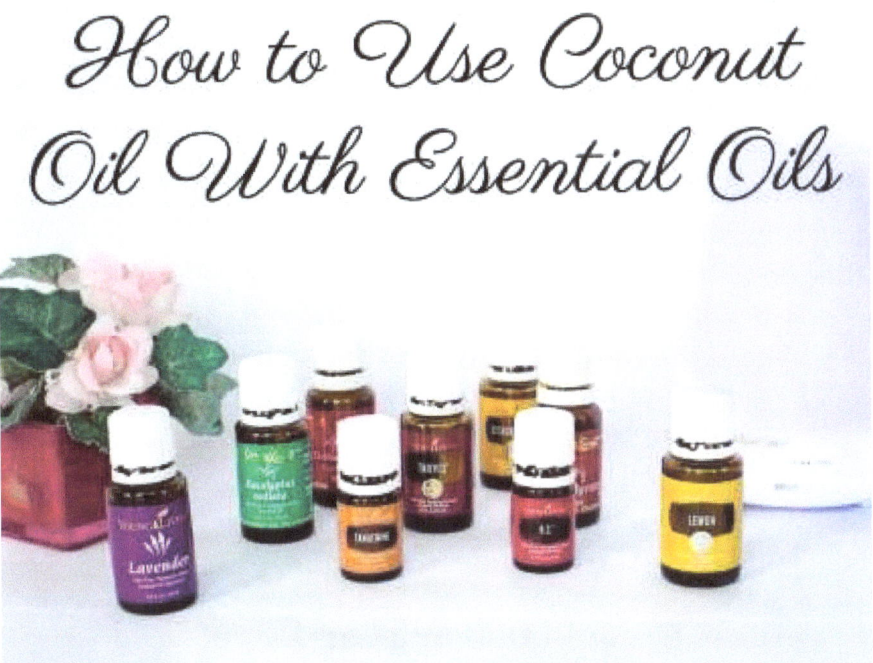

Essential oils are a great way to relax at the end of the day, help with anxiety and depression, and even reduce your stress levels. They can be used during yoga, bedtime rituals, baths, and meditation. However, you also need to combine your essential oils with a carrier oil if they are going to be applied to your skin. This is where coconut oil comes in. Here is more information about using coconut oil with essential oils.

Use Coconut Oil as a Carrier Oil

When you are using coconut oil with essential oils, you are often using it as a carrier oil. What this means is that when you apply essential oils directly to your skin, the carrier oil is mixed with the essential oil so those extracts don't irritate your skin. The problem with just rubbing in pure essential oil directly on your skin is that it can often be too harsh and lead to irritation. With carrier oils, they have a neutral scent, but they help dilute your essential oils.

It is important that you understand what oils can be used as carrier oils as well. While coconut oil is great, it isn't the only option. You can also use oils like grapeseed oil, sweet almond oil, and jojoba oil. However, you should not use cooking oils like vegetable oil and canola oil. They don't have a neutral smell and don't work good with essential oils.

Benefits of Coconut Oil For a Carrier Oil

There are two types of coconut oil you can use as a carrier oil with essential oils, including regular organic coconut oil and fractionated coconut oil. The benefits of regular coconut oil are having a solid white color, neutral smell, long shelf life, and extra moisture for your skin. If you want the oil to always be in a liquid state and absorb very well, you can also use fractionated coconut oil to mix it with your essential oils.

How to Combine it With Essential Oils

Finally, you will need to learn how to properly mix your essential oils with the coconut oil if you use it as a carrier oil. It is basically diluting the essential oils to protect your sensitive skin. It should have about 4 drop of carrier oil (coconut oil in this case) for every 1 drop of essential oil.

It is about a 20 percent dilution. Keep in mind when the essential oils are used in a bath, dilution isn't necessary.

Top Ways to Use Coconut For Pain Relief

Experiencing chronic pain is hard enough to deal with, without having to add in harsh chemicals and drugs into the mix. If you want a more natural treatment for your pain, you might want to consider using coconut oil. Take a look at how coconut oil can help with chronic pain relief.

Understand the Benefits

Before getting into how you can use coconut oil for pain relief, you should understand how exactly it helps with pain. Coconut oil is good for pain related to inflammation and joints, which is why it is perfect for conditions like arthritis and even carpal tunnel syndrome. The fatty acids that are in coconut oil make it an ideal choice when you want to help reduce inflammation in your joints and strengthen your bones. It can also increase blood circulation in the affected areas, which is great for relieving your pain.

How to Use Coconut Oil For Pain

Now for the fun part – actually applying the coconut oil! What you want to do is apply the oil directly to the areas of your body that are causing you pain. However, coconut oil usually comes in more of a solid form unless you store it in a warm environment, so you will need to liquefy it enough to where you can massage it on your aching joints and parts. With a smaller container, you can just hold it in between your hands, but with larger containers, you might need to heat them up first.

Make a Pain Relief Balm

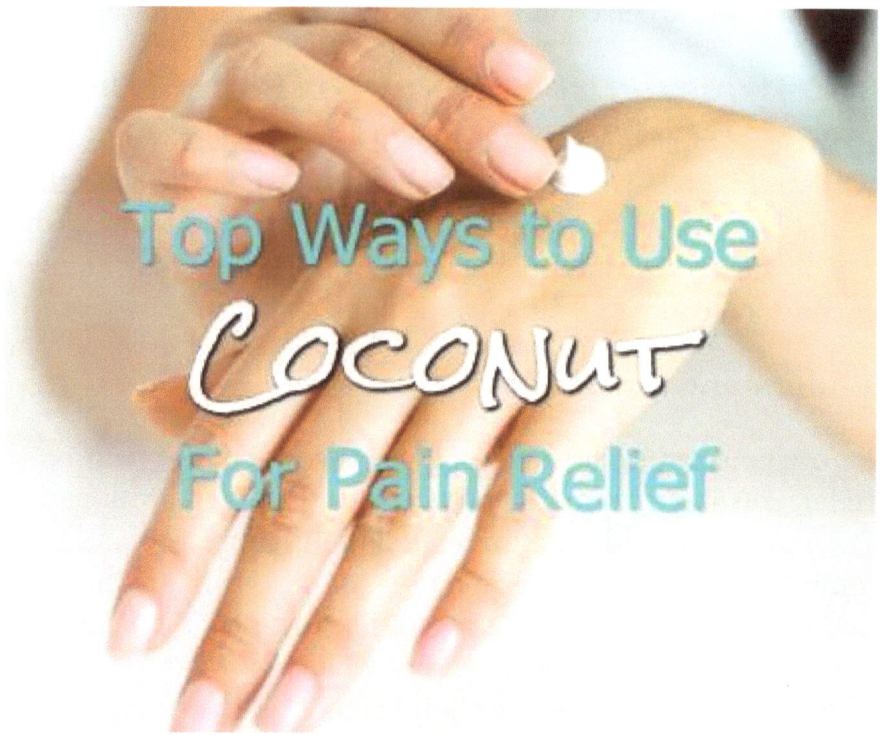

Not only can you rub the coconut oil directly on the joints or areas of your body that are hurting, but you can make your very own balm. This includes coconut oil and some other natural ingredients that are meant to help you provide more relief, without buying something at the store or having to take heavy drugs every time you are having pain. While there are a lot of different recipes, you should try to use apple cider vinegar and turmeric in the balm. The reason is because both of these provide a lot of amazing health benefits with reducing swelling and inflammation, which is perfect for arthritis and related conditions. If you have a burn on your skin that accompanies the pain, then you can also use aloe vera in the balm, which will provide some soothing power as well..

Ways to Use Coconut Oil For Tattoos

Are you interested in getting a new tattoo? If so, you will be told by the tattoo artist that you need to keep the tattoo clean and moisturized so that it heals properly. One way to do this is by using coconut oil. Take a look at these different ways to use coconut oil for your tattoos.

Moisturize a New Tattoo

One of the best uses of coconut oil for your tattoos is by moisturizing them. You are not supposed to let your new tattoo dry out when you first get it as it can be uncomfortable and affect the healing process. However, you also don't necessarily need to use the lotion recommended by the tattoo artist. Another way to keep your new tattoo properly moisturized is to use coconut oil. You do want to be careful with it and test the oil on a different area of your skin to make sure you don't have an allergic reaction. If you don't get a red and itchy patch of skin, it should be safe enough to moisturize your tattoo with.

Help Heal the Scarred Skin

After you get a tattoo, you probably have some scabs and scars that grows over the tattoo. This is temporary and just a result of the needle poking your skin to get the tattoo. Your skin bleeds during a tattoo, which then needs to repair. You can wait for this to happen naturally, or speed up the healing process a little bit by using coconut oil on your tattoos. The coconut oil has proteins that actually help to repair skin cells, which often get damaged while getting a tattoo.

Protect Your Tattoo in a Natural Way

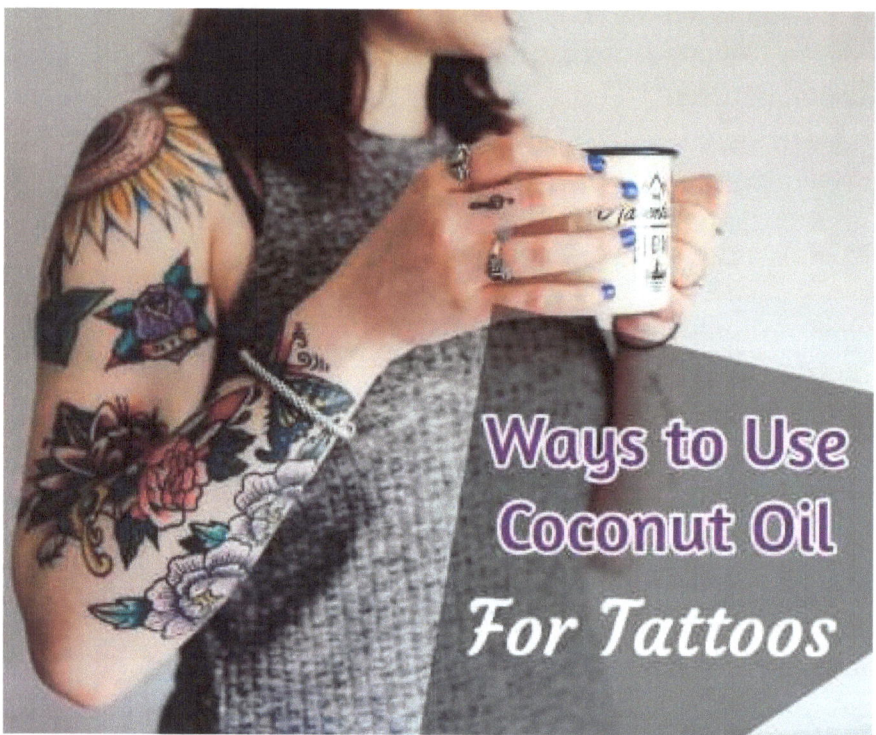

In addition to being able to keep your tattoo moisturized and helping to speed up the healing process, coconut oil can also help to protect the skin following a tattoo. Infections are not common, but they do happen if you don't take good care of your tattoo. Even with regular cleansing and moisturizing with an unscented lotion, germs and bacteria can spread. These infections are painful and sometimes hard to treat over the freshly tattooed skin. However, with coconut oil, there are proteins and fatty acids that can also work as disinfectants, helping to protect your tattoo and keep it from turning into a nasty skin infection.

Talk to your tattoo artist or doctor about using coconut oil for the purpose of helping with your tattooed skin.

Why Every Home Should Have Coconut Oil in the Bathroom

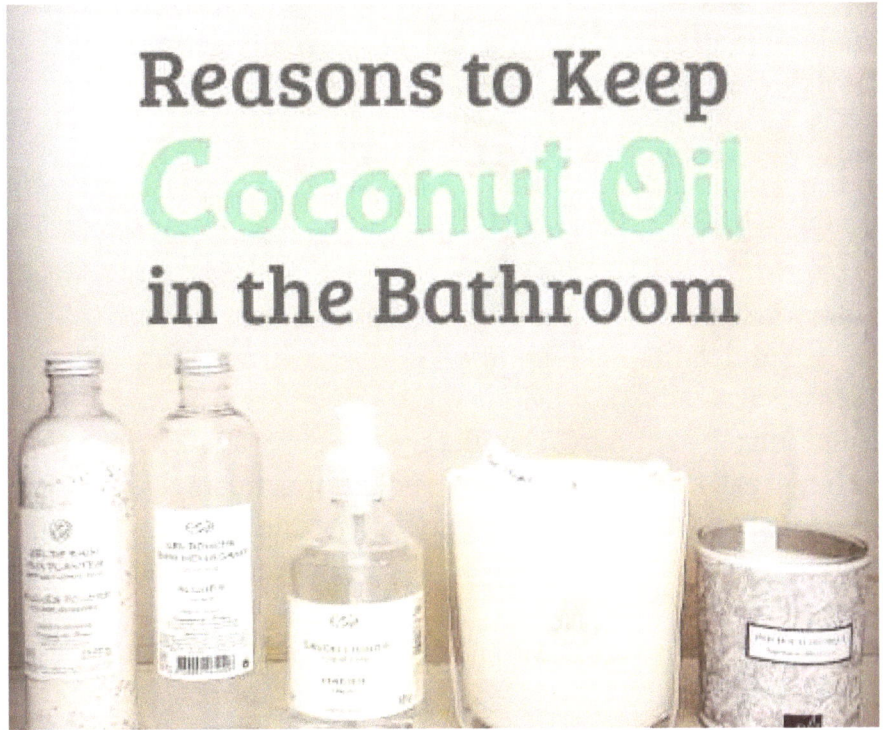

Keeping coconut oil in the home is always a good idea, since it has so many different uses for your body, hair, pets, and even pests in the home. Here are some different reasons you should always have some coconut oil in the bathroom.

You Can Use it as a Moisturizer

Here is a really simple and great reason to keep coconut oil in the bedroom. Any time you need to moisturize any part of your skin, it is safe to use coconut oil. Something you may not know is that coconut oil is safe to use on burns, cuts, and scrapes, as long as you don't have an allergic reaction to it.

This means while other lotions that are scented or have harsh ingredients can burn your skin when you have a cut in the skin, you can still use coconut oil to moisturize without making matters worse. This makes it a really good moisturizer to have on hand at all times.

It Works as a Shaving Oil

If you have trouble getting your regular shaving cream to work on your skin, or it leaves behind dry and bumpy skin afterward, then coconut oil just might be the right answer. By keeping a tub of coconut oil in the bathroom, you have easy access to it when you need to shave. You can use it in its solid form by rubbing a small amount on your face, legs, or other areas that need to be shaved, and just using your favorite razor. This not only gives you a slick and smooth surface for shaving, but the oil leaves behind soft skin afterwards that is moisturized.

Wash Your Face

Coconut oil can also be a really good facial cleanser. Since it is natural and moisturizing, it not only gets rid of dead skin cells from your face and works to remove makeup and other dirt from our face, but it will leave it well moisturized afterward. You might even find that you don't need another moisturizer after you have washed your face with it. Just make sure you mix it with water or even castor oil to dilute it a little bit, and not leave your skin oily afterward.

Clean Your Teeth With Oil Pulling

Oil pulling should not replace brushing and flossing your teeth, but it can be used in addition to normal oral health practices.

With oil pulling, you put a tablespoon of coconut oil in your warm mouth, then start swishing it around. Focus on pushing it back and forth between your teeth with your tongue, which helps to clean between your teeth and around your gum line.

Pregnancy and Newborns

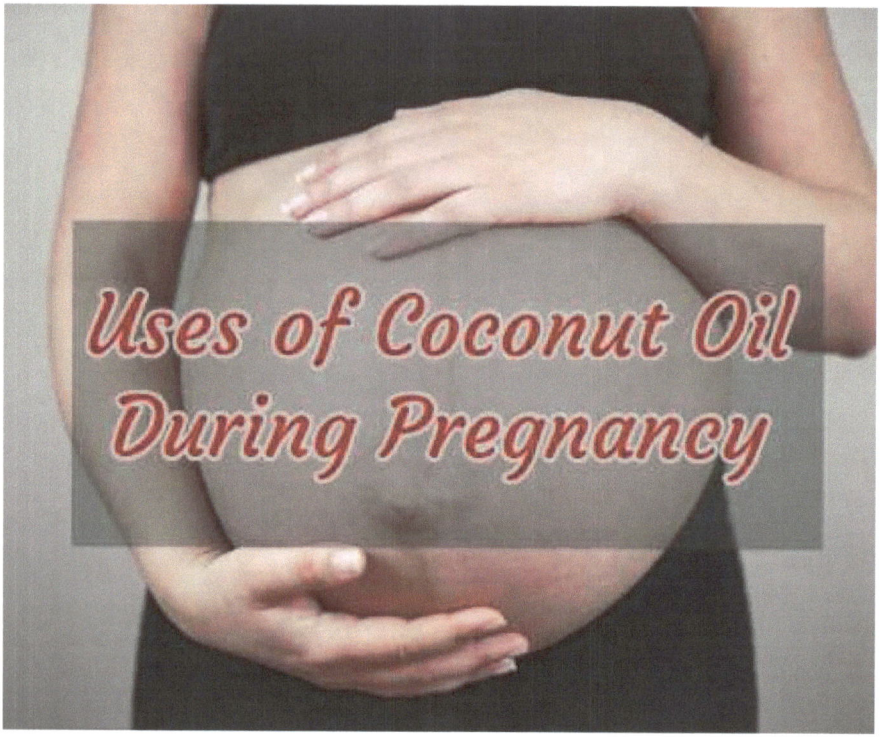

If you are currently pregnant, coconut oil is a fantastic addition to your natural health arsenal. With your doctor's permission, you can use coconut oil to benefit in the following ways.

Substitute Coconut Oil For Dairy

Many women find that they have a hard time drinking or eating anything with dairy products during pregnancy, as well as while breastfeeding. If this applies to you, then coconut oil can be a great addition to your diet.

You are able to swap out your milk and butter for coconut oil in various recipes, which is perfect if you are lactose intolerant but want certain recipes calling for dairy products. It is also good for getting more nutrients in your beverages and meals when you have your baby and your baby shows signs of having a dairy intolerance.

It is an Excellent Supplement

When you are pregnant, a simple way to use coconut oil is by using it as a supplement. There are a lot of benefits for your health in coconut oil, including help to lower your cholesterol levels and blood pressure, and protecting you against bacteria and viruses. You don't want to have to struggling with an illness during pregnancy, and your physical health is really important to ensure you have a healthy baby. So start taking a coconut oil supplement, or have a tablespoon of coconut oil every morning when you are taking your prenatal and other vitamins or supplements.

You Can Reduce Irritation

Pregnancy changes your hormone levels and causes quite a few changes in your body, and especially your skin. That might include getting dry and cracked skin, sometimes with red and irritating rashes. Coconut oil can soothe your skin to reduce itchiness, get rid of red patches, and help with those dry areas of skin. You can rub it on any itchy or dry areas of skin during pregnancy, then also use it after you have the baby to apply on your cracked nipples while breastfeeding.

Ease Your Side Effects

Don't forget that a lot of your other pregnancy side effects can get relief by using coconut oil. For example, adding a little coconut oil to your food or drinks each day can help with digestion and bacteria in your esophagus. This can help to reduce morning sickness, heartburn, and nausea that are common during pregnancy. You can also make a natural headache balm to use for relieving your headaches, since you can't take regular pain killers while you are pregnant.

Safety Tips For Using Coconut Oil On Newborns

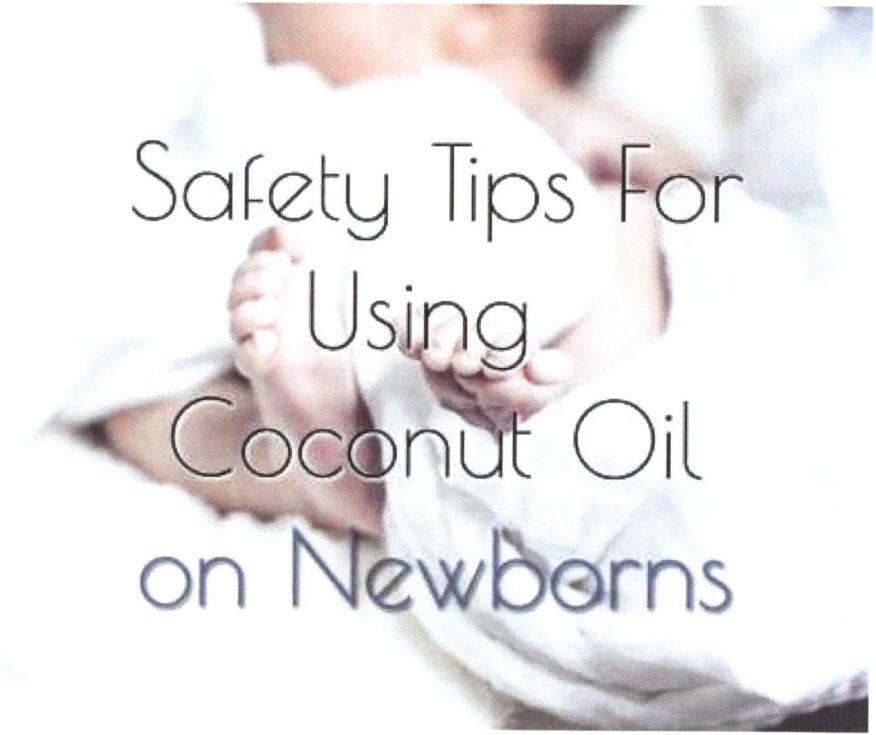

Coconut oil is very safe to use for most people, except for those who have an allergic reaction to it. Even young children and babies can benefit from coconut oil for things like minor cuts and scrapes, but you need to be extra careful. Here are some tips for using it safely on your newborn or infant.

Test the Oil First

Before you start using coconut oil on your newborn baby, after talking to your doctor, make sure you have tested it on a small area of skin. Use a very small amount of the coconut oil, making sure it is only organic and all-natural virgin coconut oil. Don't warm it up to scalding, only enough to get it a little more malleable. Rub a small amount on a very small section of skin, then wait a few minutes to see if there is a reaction. If your baby starts crying, or you notice redness or other signs of irritation, do not use it on your baby. While it is safe for most people, some have an allergic reaction to it.

Use the Right Type of Oil

You also need to make sure you are using coconut oil that is safest and most natural for your newborn baby. Don't just get any type of coconut oil without looking at both the label and the ingredients list. This puts you at risk of getting coconut oil with additives, preservatives, or that has gone through a chemical process. You want your baby to have the most natural form, which means looking for raw, organic coconut oil that is virgin or extra virgin, and is unrefined, not refined. This will be the most natural coconut oil possible for your baby.

Be Careful With Diaper Rash

Coconut oil is often recommended to use on diaper rash, but you need to be careful. This is when using only organic, extra virgin coconut oil with nothing added comes in handy. Only use a very small amount, and ask your pediatrician before you use it. They may have noticed negative reactions with coconut oil if you used it for other purposes, and may suggest you not use it. You can also make your own natural baby wipes with soft microfiber cloths and coconut oil to prevent the diaper rashes from forming in the first place.

Most babies can tolerate coconut oil with no trouble, but always test it first and ensure it is not warm after you have melted it.

Around the House

3 Natural Stain Removers

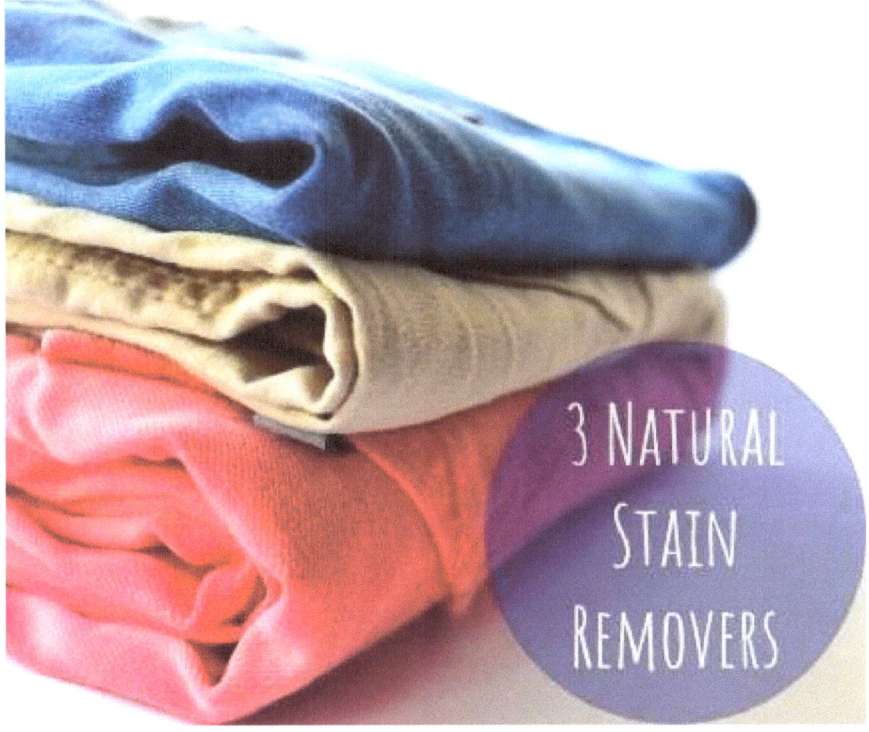

If you have a stain on your carpet, rug, or clothing, you might be trying to use a store-bought product to remove the stain. Not only are these not always the most effective method, but they often contain harsh ingredients you might not want on your body or in your home. A better option is to turn to natural stain removers, such as those listed here.

Basic Stain Remover Spray

This first natural stain remover only contains a few simple ingredients in order to help you get rid of stains in clothing or other fabrics without using any harsh ingredients. You can put the finished mixture in a spray bottle and keep it in your laundry room. Spray stains before putting clothes or linens in the washer, and it should work great. For the simplest recipe, you just need some natural soap, such as Dr. Bronners Sal Suds, water, and coconut oil, plus a spray bottle. Combine the ingredients in the bottle, then spray it on the stains before washing.

Other Ingredients to Use

You can also use a variety of other natural ingredients to make your own stain remover spray. You may find some type of secret combination that works best for you and want to keep it a secret, or you can find a combination that people often like to use. Here are some of the best options for natural ingredients when talking about a stain remover:

- Baking Soda

- Vinegar

- Hydrogen Peroxide

- Natural Soap

- Coconut Oil

- Lemon Juice

- Oxygen Bleach

When you are putting together your very own natural stain remover, make sure you are careful about it and that you don't test it on a large piece of fabric or clothing. Test it on something like a towel first to make sure it doesn't change the color of the material or cause other bad reactions.

How to Use Your Coconut Oil Stain Remover

Once you have made your natural stain remover with coconut oil and other natural ingredients, make sure you never rub the stain. Whether it is in carpet, your clothing, or linens, blotting should always be done. If you catch the stain following a spill when it is wet, blot it dry with paper towels first. You can then spray the stain and blot it once more. The only exception is when it is on clothing you are about to put in the washer. You can apply the stain remover, let it sit for a few minutes, then put it in the washer.

Pest Control Tips: Use Coconut Oil For Pests

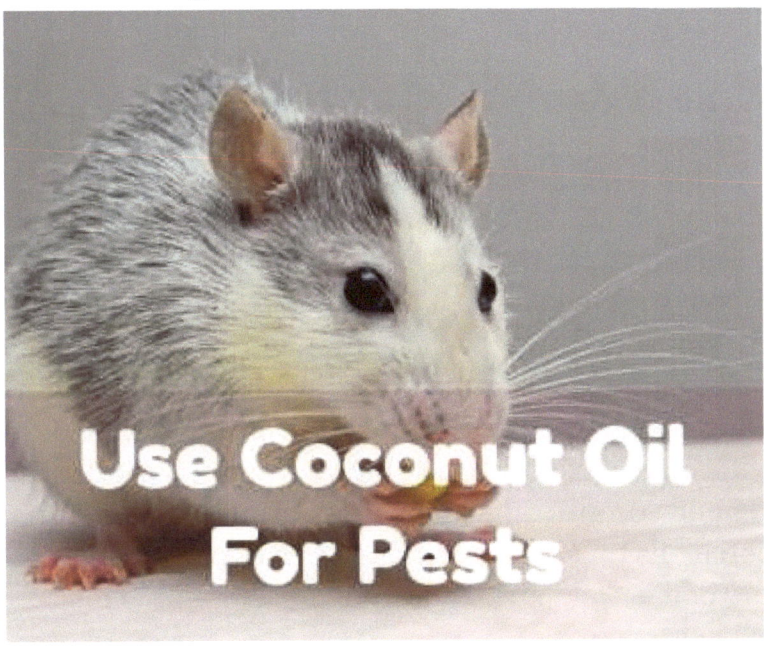

Many people use coconut oil for things like soft hair and treating cuts and scrapes on the skin, but don't forget it also has a lot of uses right in your home. For example, you can use coconut oil to help with pests in your home. Here are some pest control tips for using coconut oil at home.

Get Better Control of Spiders

If you have a spider problem in your home, which is one of the most common pests people have to deal with, then you can use coconut oil as a natural pest repellent. There are some different ways to do this, depending on what ingredients you want to mix it with and whether it is being used indoors or outdoors. For example, if you have cobwebs in your home and want to get rid of the spiders, you can mix vinegar with coconut oil into a spray bottle, then spray all the cobwebs. The spiders will not return to those areas. Outdoors, you can also use this similar type of mixture and spray trees, plants, and piles of cardboard or boxes in the garage where you tend to find the spiders most often.

Basic Bug Balm

This recipe is going to help you make a small container of bug balm, which can be used on most pests in your home. This is going to be a soft bug balm, which is actually used on your body, not to kill pests. It is going to help keep the bugs away from your skin to avoid getting bites. You can use it at home on summer days when bugs inside are more common, or bring it with you on hikes and during other outdoor activities. To make the bug balm, you want to combine shea butter and coconut oil with beeswax granules. You then use essential oils that bugs don't like, such as citronella, cedarwood, eucalyptus, and lemongrass essential oils.

Find Relief From Bug Bites

Another way that coconut oil helps with pests in the home is not by killing the bugs, but by relieving your skin if you get a bite or sting. For example, if you have bed bugs, they can go crazy on your skin, leading to bad bites and really itchy skin. The same thing happens when spiders and other bugs bite you at night. You can use coconut oil to rub on your skin and find relief from the itching.

Final Thoughts

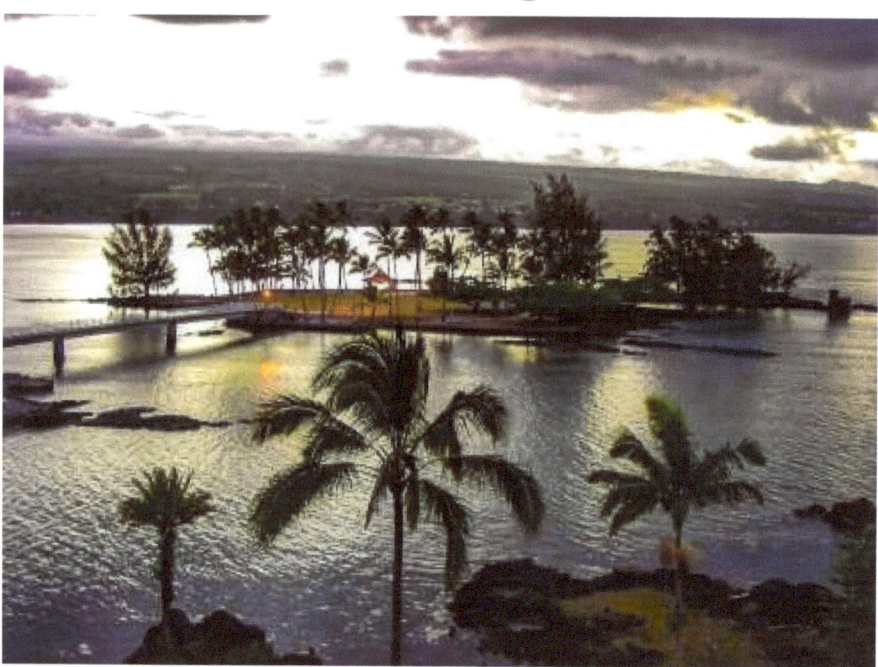

Coconut oil is a plant-based saturated fat that is very healthy for you inside and out. It promotes clear, wrinkle free skin and protects against sunburn and skin cancer. Originally lumped together with animal–based saturated fats and avoided, it actually has none of their bad properties. Instead it is gaining in reputation and popularity extremely fast.

A functional food, it is rich in fiber, vitamins and minerals. The coconut palm tree is referred to as the "tree of life" because, besides its food value, so many things are made from it and it can be used on the human body with many benefits. Coconut oil is squeezed from the "meat" of the coconut and the best type is organic cold pressed extra virgin coconut oil.

Coconut oil is an easily digested fat. It is composed of medium chain fatty acids, which go straight to the liver and are turned into energy. This is great news for people who have had their gall bladder removed, since it is needed to digest long chain fatty acids found in animal fats but not the MCFAs in coconut oil.

Coconut oil contains high amounts of lauric acid that is the same as found in mother's milk, the only other source of sufficient levels and one of the reasons for breastfeeding benefits in infants and their low incidence of disease in later life.

Coconut oil is actually 50% lauric acid. Lauric acid is transformed by the body into monolaurin.

That, along with the capric and caprylic acids also in coconut oil, has antimicrobial, antiviral, antifungal and anti-protozoal properties. It is a highly effective treatment for candida albicans and targets bacterial infections and many other diseases. Researchers are eyeing it for treatment in HIV/Aids.

You can get a small amount of lauric acid from dried coconut meat and coconut milk, but the oil contains almost four times that amount. You can take about 3 tablespoons of coconut oil daily. You can just eat it off a spoon, use it when frying your meals, or put it in smoothies. That amount will protect you from viruses and bacteria as well as help your skin from the inside. It will also boost your metabolism and help you burn body fat.

The only side effect when you start using coconut oil is if you have been on a low fat diet, you may experience diarrhea until you become used to taking it. Improve this by taking smaller doses spread out over the course of the day.

Other Relevant Books by This Author

If you would like to read more relevant books about this topic, here is a list of the Amazon Paperback links, titles and descriptions from this author:

https://www.amazon.com/Energy-Supercharge-Your-Body-More/dp/1520732406

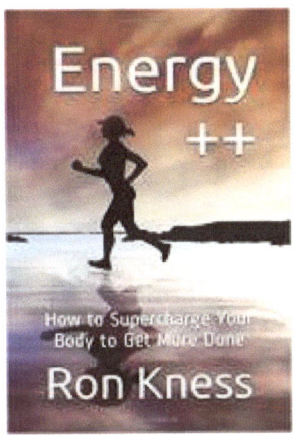

Energy ++: How to Supercharge Your Body to Get More Done

We want to be in control of our body's energy management program.

We also want to be empowered to have more energy to accomplish more each day ... and with better results. And we want to know how to supercharge our body to get more done each day!

We can achieve ALL of these goals with the newest release from Ron Kness called *Energy ++.*

Based on these exciting teachings, you will learn about all the dramatic benefits of creating more energy through healthy eating and using a unique three-event exercise program called QUICK.

This book is built around a very clear, concept: have energy left at the end of the work day to spend with family and friends. It's not just about getting more done each day. Having great productivity both at home and at work is linked to managing time along with energy.

This is because the two go hand-in-hand in regard to productivity. In this book, we look at all of the ways you can improve your own productivity both at home and at work, starting with knowing what things to add to your life and what to cut out.

This book will also look at the many other steps that can be taken to support this goal, from eating healthy nutritious food and exercising to living a healthy lifestyle by cutting out unhealthy habits like smoking. The choices you make about eating and exercising have an impact on the amount of energy you have both at home and at work.

In *Energy ++,* we'll cover all the bases, giving you everything you need to know to have the energy to do everything you want to do each day.

https://www.amazon.com/TLC-Diet-Transformation-Cholesterol-Transform/dp/1520705549

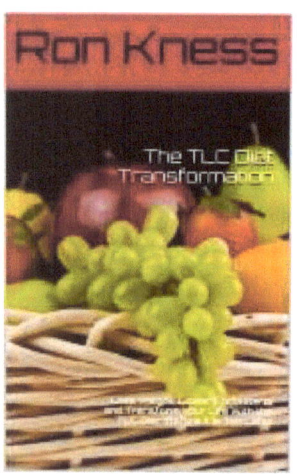

The TLC Diet Transformation: Lose Weight, Lower Cholesterol and Transform Your Life With the TLC Diet (Before It Is Too Late)!

Discover the diet plan that has taken the world by storm and been voted one of the best diets of 2017!"

Read on to find out exactly how you can change your life by following a simple diet that anyone can do... with phenomenal results. Obesity is on the rise! The state of obesity in the world today is a concern for all governments ... especially those in developed countries and with this comes the rise of hypertension and high cholesterol levels.

Despite the efforts governments have taken, the epidemic seems to become more serious. It affects both children as well as adults. The main reason for the growth of this epidemic is lack of proper diet among the people. Most of the people have limited physical exercises as children spend a lot of time playing video and internet games or watching television.

Although this is a big epidemic, there is a solution... Introducing the *TLC Diet Transformation*.

It can help you lose weight, lower your cholesterol and transform your life into one of a healthy lifestyle. However, unlike most other diets, the TLC is not a deprivation diet. The TLC diet is among the most established diets for the natural management of cholesterol. It has been formulated based on scientific evidences conducted by experts in the field of medicine. Many individuals are currently using the diet as recommended by their physicians to achieve good cholesterol levels & regulated blood pressure levels.

In my book *The TLC Diet Transformation*, here is exactly what you get: • Learn Exactly What The TLC Diet Is • Discover The Key To Properly Planning Your TLC Diet • Practical Advice On The Best Foods To Eat On The TLC Diet • How To Shop Smart And Buy Foods That Are Nutritionally Sound • Sample Recipes & Tips To Start Today • And Much, Much More..

This powerful guide will provide you with all the necessary information to easily transition you into living a healthy lifestyle and finally achieve your dream of dropping cholesterol and stopping hypertension in its tracks.

So make the choice today. If you need to drop cholesterol and curb hypertension, this guide could be the first step in the journey towards the new healthier you.

https://www.amazon.com/Secrets-Healthy-Lifestyle-Changes-Make/dp/1542418631

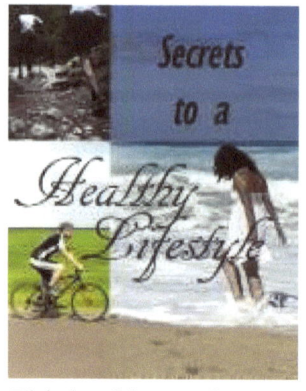

Secrets to a Healthy Lifestyle: 7 Lifestyle Changes To Make This Year the Best Yet

Along with a New Year comes the opportunity to let go of the past and start fresh and anew. It's a perfect time to get serious about getting healthy. Don't think of it as a new year's resolution.

Think of it as a brand-new start on your life. Out with the old, and in with the new. What's more is that it's not as difficult as you think.

You can have less stress with a few simple daily actions, eat better by adding in more healthy food and get healthier by exercising more without feeling like it's so much work. In addition, just a few money and time management, and unhealthy habit changes will make all the difference in your life.

Finally, you'll have more time for more fun without spending tons of money. You're going to feel so much better with just a few specific changes, that you'll have the very best year you've ever had. Turn off electronics, head for a walk in the park, have a picnic, then go grocery shopping leisurely.

Make fun a priority in your life and you'll naturally be healthier, happier and have an amazing year, every year.

About the Author

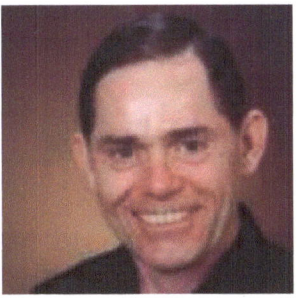

I have published over 125 books on Amazon for Kindle, CreateSpace and other publishing platforms.

While most of my books are on health and fitness in general, as I age (now 65) at the time of this writing) my topics of interest are geared toward aging baby boomers and older.

Besides my own writing, I also ghostwrite ebooks, books, reports, articles, blogs and do Kindle conversions for clients on a variety of topics.

Today my wife and I are retired from our careers and live in Gold Canyon, AZ. I now write as a retirement business where you'll find me happily sitting in my office typing away on my laptop as I work on my next book or ghostwriting project . . . that is if we are not traveling on a cruise ship - our new-found mode of travel.

www.ingramcontent.com/pod-product-compliance
Lightning Source LLC
Chambersburg PA
CBHW050821290526

45792CB00001B/215